# MEDICAL EQUIPMENT
## AND
# SUPPLY BUSINESS

# MEDICAL EQUIPMENT
# AND
# SUPPLY BUSINESS

*Your Multi Billion Dollar Guide to Start-Up*

Medical Equipment/Supply

**A STEP BY STEP GUIDE TO START-UP**

**In Business for Life**

YOUR HOW TO GUIDE TO BUSINESS START-UP

# J.S. SPRATLEY

| Library of Congress Control Number: | | 2012905241 |
|---|---|---|
| ISBN: | Hardcover | 978-1-4691-8721-1 |
| | Softcover | 978-1-4691-8720-4 |
| | Ebook | 978-1-4691-8722-8 |

**To order additional copies of this book, contact:**
Xlibris Corporation
1-888-795-4274
www.Xlibris.com
Orders@Xlibris.com
113504

# ABOUT THE AUTHOR

I first started in the medical field in the early 80's. I started out as a volunteer in a local hospital, fresh out of high school and out of work. I decided to volunteer myself for the good of others. While volunteering my service for about six months at a local hospital I was offered a job as an orderly. While of course I was very happy to have a job with my own money coming in. I was not satisfied with being in this position. I knew I would not make a career of this job.

Coming in to work one evening I notice on the job board a position posted for a Respiratory Therapist. Having been working in the hospital I would meet other employees, and the director of Respiratory Therapy was one whom I had the pleasure to have met. When I went up to the director's office (with job posting in hand) I was no stranger to him. I informed him that I wanted to apply for the position of Respiratory Therapist. The director informed me that I would need to go to school to obtain my Respiratory Therapy credentials. To make this long story short I went to school and obtained my certification as a Respiratory Therapist licensed to practice Respiratory Therapy for the state of Virginia. Working as a Respiratory Therapist for about ten years I decided to start my own Respiratory Homecare Company. Having Three Thousand Dollars in hand, which I saved over a few years I knew I was determined to me this money work for me. While still maintaining my full time job I started operating my homecare company on a part time base. I maintained both jobs for about eight years before I had to make the choice to do just one or the other. I chose to leave the hospital and make my homecare business my full time career. Feeling very apprehensive about leaving the hospital (mainly the security of a full time job and the benefits) I took the plunge and did it. With everything relying on me now, to make this business work I knew I had to do more. This is when I added the medical equipment and supplies to my business. Seeing the consistent need for these products I knew that this would boost my profits. I started out providing equipment and supplies that I was familiar with. I started with five products (Gloves. Wipes, Biohazard/Trash Bags, Wheelchairs, and Crutches) and within Three Months I was up to ten products, and within a year I was able to supply my customers with almost whatever they needed. I was supplying over one hundred twenty different products, and if I did not have it, my customer never knew that I didn't have it, because I would make it a point to get it.

I recently sold my company and have semi-retired (and by the way did I mention that I operated this company alone, one person). My goal now is to educate those that have very little to no knowledge in the way of starting and operating a successful medical equipment and supply business. I want to educate those who are like I was when I first started (with no knowledge of business), and with even less start-up money that I had when I started. My intent is to be an advocate for those people. With this easy to understand, step by step, right to the point book that I have prepared just for the purpose of those wanting to start a very profitable business, and with a very minimum start-up of less than Three hundred Dollars.

The medical equipment and supply business has been a great business for me. It has given me the opportunity to travel, meet new people, and enjoy the independent life that I often dreamed of. The opportunity for growth in this business is endless. There is no limit to how much you can grow this very profitable business.

With over thirty years in the medical field I have seen many changes some bad, but mostly good. I wrote this book for those with not a lot of upfront money, for those with no knowledge of medical equipment and supply, for those with little knowledge of how to start up a business, and for those who will not have valuable information (such as this) without paying thousands of dollars for a lot of books and tape that don't really tell them nothing. It has been very exciting for me to have put this information down in writing, knowing that it will be for the benefit and a life style change for its readers.

# MEDICAL EQUIPMENT AND SUPPLY BUSINESS

It is a fact that the population of people is living longer. New medical technology and science today have extended the lives of the human population by 5-10 years. With this new extended lifespan, come new extended problems, related to medical health issues.

That is where the business of medicine comes in, and with that comes more medical care, which requires more medical equipment and supplies. The medical equipment and supply business as of today is a multi-billion dollar a year business nationally (that does not include international)

The medical equipment and supply business is a business that has been proven to withstand the hard economic times that we are in the midst of. This is a business that will never fold. The potential for growth with this business has no limits. One can work this medical supply business as much or as little as is needed. With the Federal, State, and Local Governments being mandated to use more small businesses (like yours) to provide them with services and products, this is the perfect time to start this very profitable business, and be a part of this medical equipment and supply business success.

This is a business that you can run from the comfort of your home (in a spare room) or right from your kitchen table. There is no stocking of any equipment or supplies (unless you choose to).

Through the direction of this book you will be on your way to operating your own medical equipment and Supply Company and having your portion of this multi-billion dollar industry.

The medical equipment and supply industry is, and will be around forever. This is not a get rich quick scam. You will have to sell your business to your potential customer. With the medical equipment and supply business you can now live the life that you have dreamed of for so long.

# CONTENTS

# LOCATE MY RESOURCES

(These areas may vary from state to state)

*Zoning Requirement:* Contact your local city/county administration Offices (Clerk's office)

*Business Name:* Contact your local city/county administration office (Clerk's office)

*Business License:* Contact your local city/county administration office (Business License Division)

*Tax ID Number/Employer ID Number (EIN):* Go online @ *www.IRS. GOV/einform* and apply

*Taxes:* (State and Local) Contact your state department of taxation for state Taxes and the department of revenue for your city/county taxes

*Business Banking:* Contact your favorite bank for all your business needs (Compare rates for business checking accounts for the best deal)

*What Other License(s) Do I Need:* See this section of the book?

*Privacy Act:* (HIPAA.gov)

*Business Insurance:* Contact local insurance companies in your area or perform an online search using Google for business insurance

**Business Tools:** (business phone/fax, computer, website) Contact local offices supply, online stores, department stores, etc.

**Business Material:** (Business cards/fliers) Contact your local printing company, office supply store, or using your computer do it yourself online

**Method of Payment:** (Credit card, Checks, Cash) Contact you bank, credit union, or financial institution merchant service

Department to sign your business up to accept credit cards

**Recordkeeping/Bookkeeping:** Go to local office supply store or department store to purchase a bookkeeping journal or go online

To order QuickBooks software (QuickBooks has a support staff for questions which is very user friendly

**Business Plan:** Go online and Google "sample business plan" for a sample of how to plan for your business success

**Hire Employees:** This is at your own Choice (Make sure your business needs warrant an employee.

**Home Based Business:** Your choice of operating from home or rent/own a location elsewhere

**Press Release:** Contact local newspaper

**Sales Representative:** Contact your medical supply company

**Who Do I Sell To and What Do I Say?** See this section of the book

**What Can I Sell?** See this section of the book?

*Drop Shipping:* Contact your medical supply company's sales rep.

*Medical Supplier/Distributor Companies* (Products Provided)

*Medical Supplier/Distributor Companies* (Phone List)

*Medical Supplier/Distributor Companies* (Website)

*Helpful Sites:* See this section of the book

*Calculation of your start-up costs*

*Did You Remember:* (Getting started checklist) See this section of the book

*Medical Glove Market Research:*

# ZONING REQUIREMENTS

(Contact local city/county administration offices)

The first step in starting your business is to check to see if you can operate that business from your home or any other location. This is done by contacting your local city or county administration/Government office. This process may vary from state to state, (while some may require this, others may not) but your Government office officials will know.

This is an easy process, which normally takes about 5-10 minutes to complete. This is done to protect the policies of some communities that have rules and regulations of what you can and cannot have in certain neighborhoods. These rules would apply to a business that would have customers or employees coming and going on a regular base from the residence, or having advertising signs posted outside the residence. This is something that you wouldn't have to do, so you should not have to worry about whether or not you will be approved.

# REGISTERING BUSINESS NAME

(Contact local city/county clerk's office)
(This may vary from state to state)

Your next step is to register your business name. This process is done to allow for the use of your business name, if not already in use. You would (in most cities or counties) put your business name into a computer data base, which would then search to match your business name to any other business with that same name. If a match is found, you would then have to choose another name for your business. However, if no match is found for the name that you are using, then you are clear to use the business name you have chosen.

When choosing a name for your business, choose a name that reflects what you are doing. If for instance, one should see your business name they would know at that point exactly what it is that you do. Example; (USA medical equipment and supply sales). You can tell by this business name that they sell medical equipment and supplies. Do not let your potential customer guess at what your business does.

# BUSINESS LICENSE

(Contact local city/county administration offices)
(This may vary from state to state)

This next step gives you the right to conduct your business. This is a simple process, but with different variations from state to state. You would apply for your business license at your local city or county administration/ government offices. Some cities/counties will allow you to apply online for your business license. There is no fee to apply, however at the time of applying you will be asked how much do you anticipate on making with the business in the year that you are applying. For example, if you apply for your business license in June 2011 they would want to know your gross income for the remaining months of 2011. Here is the thing, no one ever knows what they're income will be, so you would come up with a figure (keep it low) of what you think you will gross. I would suggest using $100. 00 as your anticipated gross income and no tax would be accessed at that point.

Keep in mind that you will be taxed on the income you receive during that year when it comes to your yearly renewal of your business license.

# WHAT OTHER LICENSE(S) DO I NEED

(Contact the Board of Pharmacy)

As a medical equipment and supply provider, you can provide some drugs under your business. Although you may or may not want to provide drugs the board of pharmacy looks at it as you can. Each board may vary in its rules and regulations on having such a license, so it is necessary to contact your State Board of Pharmacy for your medical equipment and supply license requirements.

The Board of Pharmacy is a regulatory organization for the use of drugs and medical equipment. There is a basic application process (fairly simple) along with a yearly fee that also varies from state to state.

Upon approval by the board and the payment of the fee, the board will issue you a license, which is renewed each year.

# TAX ID/EMPLOYERS IDENTIFICATION NUMBER (EIN)

### (Contact Internal Revenue Services, IRS.GOV)

This number is used to identify your business by the Internal Revenue Service (IRS). It can also be used when opening business bank accounts, applying for business license, and filing your tax returns. You can apply for and obtain this number through the IRS website at IRS.GOV/EINFORM (click on apply for an employer identification number online) then click (apply online now). This is a very simple process and when applying online you will receive your number right away. This number is very important because it separates your business affairs from your personal affairs, something that you must keep separate. (It's also the number used to pay your Federal taxes)

In the event that you do not have this number, and you are ready to move forward with starting the necessary paperwork to get your business started you may use your social security number in its place, but you must obtain this number as soon as possible.

# **TAXES** (State, Local)

(State: Contact Dept. of Taxation)
(Local: Contact Dept. of Revenue)

**State:** You must register your business with the Department of Taxation so that sales and income tax can be collected, if applicable. In some cases businesses are exempt from paying sales tax, and the medical supply business is one that can be tax exempt. You will need to complete an application to be tax exempt, and upon approval you will receive a tax exempt number. This number gives your business the right to not have any sales taxes taken when making a purchase for your business. You will need to have this number when applying for an account with your medical supply distributors; it will be your responsibilities to let your sales Rep. know that you are tax exempt so that no tax on the products that you purchase will be taken.

**Local:** You must register your business with the department of revenue or city/county tax collector office. This tax is imposed in order to allow you to operate a business in the city or county in which your business is located. This tax rate varies, depending on what type of business, the number of employees, and business equipment and supplies owned. With your business you won't have any equipment/supplies that you own, nor will you have any employees (unless you choose to) and the medical supply business is not a high risk business that requires a high tax rate, so don't worry, your business is good to go.

# BUSINESS BANKING

### (Shop Around for Bank or Credit Union)

When choosing a bank or credit union to handle your business banking needs, look for one that offers a bundle package (as I call it). Choose one that can offer your business great interest rates on your money, merchant services (credit card processing), free checking, online banking and bill pay, etc. Do not combine your personal banking with your business banking this must be kept separate. When opening your business banking account you will need to have your business license, tax ID number (EIN) or Social Security Number (SSN), and personal identification (such as drivers license, etc.).

# BUSINESS INSURANCE

(Contact Local Agents, or go online to get Quotes)

This is based on your own personal preference of which insurance company to use. I have always used Pharmacist Mutual (who specializes in medical equipment coverage) for my business insurance needs. However, you can find business insurance companies online at Google (type in) IIABA (Independent Insurance Agents and Brokers of America). When seeking insurance ask about business property insurance, which protects all your workplace property.

# BUSINESS TOOLS
## (Computer/Printer, Phone/Fax, Website)
### (Contact your Office Supply Store, Department Store, etc.)

This is possibly the most important part of your business, because it gives your customers the means of contacting your business for products.

**Computer/Printer:** Being that many people have computers already, this is an expense that you do not have to have. However, I would suggest that you get a laptop computer or some other system that you can carry around with you. It would be as though you are carrying your office around with you, which is good because you would have everything there if you are out and get a call for an order, which has happened to me on many occasions. Your printer should be the all-in-one printer which has fax/phone and copying capabilities. Contact your office supply or department stores for the systems of your choice.

**Phone:** Although a landline phone is good, a cell phone for your business use is just as good. In my opinion it is better, because you have the capability to carry your phone with you and not miss those all important call (orders), which means more business. If possible and if your budget allows it, get the cell phone with internet/email capabilities, because some orders will be sent through your email. Contact your cell phone service provider.

**Fax:** Another avenue that your orders will be sent through is the fax. This is a must have in the medical supply sales business. Before, you would need to have a stationery fax machine connected to a phone line. Those days are over, I have found "efax" to be all that I needed to have my fax sent to me directly to my email, and I can send return faxes right from my computer. Contact efax online at efax.com it is well worth the very inexpensive cost.

**Website:** A website is a great selling tool and some companies that you will deal with will require you to have a website. This will allow them to view your products instead of calling each time to find out what you have. With that in mind I would suggest that you get a website for your business. I have used Intuit.com to build my own website with step by step instructions on how to do it, or you can have them build it for you. Through Intuit.com you are given the capability to set up payment through your website, so your customers can order right from your website, and a confirmation will be sent to you through your email notifying you of the order. Another site that will help with building your website is "Yola," Go online and Google Yola.

Another resource for all of your business tools needs is a website called: onebox.com

# BUSINESS MATERIALS
## (Business Cards/Fliers)
### (Contact Print Company, or Office supply Store)

**Business Cards/Fliers:** Business cards and fliers give your customers a glance of what your business has to offer and your contact information. These are good selling materials, but it only gives your customer a brief look at what your business has, and not the full picture. In the medical supply business you are not going to find many who need medical supplies looking at a flier to make their choice in what supplies they need. Most, already know what they need.

Hospitals or doctors' offices already know what their needs are. This is an area that should not take priority in your selling point, particularly with the fliers. The business cards are great and you can't give out enough of them, so pass them out to everyone. In an effort to keep your cost down you can go online to "free business cards" and make your own business cards for free. This site will allow you to use a template to design your cards.

# METHOD OF PAYMENT
## (Credit Card, Check, Cash)

(Contact your bank or Pay Pal Merchant Service)

Accepting payment from your customers is what will keep your business thriving. Having your business set to accept payment from your customers in any form is a must. The major portion of your customers will be paying by credit cards. Contact your bank's merchant service department to discuss being setup to provide this credit card service to your customers. However, it is very important to shop around when it comes to this service, because there is a fee to use this service, and it varies depending on the institution that you will be dealing with. That is why I chose Pay Pal Merchant services. There is no monthly fee, you only pay per transaction, and their site is 100% secure.

You must have your business bank account setup before you can use this service. This is done completely online, which was great for me because I could run my transactions whenever and wherever I was. When choosing whatever merchant service that you go with, be sure that you can accept checks with that service. A small portion of your customers will pay by check, and an even smaller portion will pay with cash. However you are paid, be ready and able to accept that payment.

# RECORDKEEPING/BOOKKEEPING

First, find yourself recordkeeping software, or a journal. I used Quick-books software in my business, which worked great for me, and it did all my calculations for me at year end. However in an effort to conserve your business startup costs buying a recordkeeping journal from your local department store's office supply section would work just as good for a fraction of the cost? It is very important to keep your business recordkeeping completely separate from your personal records.

Your recordkeeping/bookkeeping is to keep track of your business financials, such as Payroll, Income, Expenses; it acts as a database for all your business transactions.

# BUSINESS PLAN

## (Google: Sample Business Plans)

This is a laid out plan by you, as to how you will operate your business.

This is like a roadmap to your business survival, mapping out and figuring out the ups and down associated with operating a business.

This is a good tool to have, but is not always necessary. If you were trying to obtain a loan for the start-up of your business it will be a must to have a business plan in hand. Banks and other lending institutions will not even talk to you regarding a loan if you don't have a business plan. In your plan you need to ask question such as, who are your competitors, how is your business better or different than theirs, how will you maintain financially during these hard economic times, etc. These are questions that should be covered in your business plan. Go online and Google "Sample Business Plans" for sample of how business plans are written.

# HIRING EMPLOYEES

If you choose to hire employees, that is fine, but keep in mind that this is an expense that is not necessary. With the medical supply business, this can be a one person business. Hiring employees maybe something to consider in the future, but now, just starting your business, it is not necessary.

# HOME BASED BUSINESS

Set up a part of your home to operate your business, a spare bedroom, garage, or right at your kitchen table. This business only requires a small area to handle office administration duties, a place where you can setup your computer, printer/fax, and file cabinet to keep your files.

Having your business run from your home has many advantages, such as, it gives you tax deductions, there is no driving to your work destination; there is no additional rent for an office space outside your home. This is a great way to save on your start-up costs.

However, if you choose to have your businesses setup at a location other than your home that is fine. Keep in mind that you are just starting your business and an expense like rent can set you back financially. You will be locked in to pay rent for at least a year, and if for some reason you choose not to maintain the business you will still be obligated to pay rent. However, many business owners use a UPS store address so as not to use their personal home address.

# PRIVACY ACT

## (Online @ HIPAA.gov)

As a medical equipment and supply provider, you will sometimes come across patient information. This information is treated with strict confidentiality and no person shall disclose any information related to that patient.

The governing board that oversees these regulations and enforces it is the Health Insurance Portability and Accountability Act (HIPAA). Violation of these regulations will result in a fine of not less than $ 250,000.

You can find these regulations at hipaa.gov and click (health information privacy-united states department of health) this is just for your reading, but the rules must be followed to the letter.

# PRESS RELEASE

## (Contact Local Paper and Online Distribution Service)

If you are starting a new business, or reopening another business in an area, most newspaper companies and online distributing services offer FREE press releases, which allow you to post your new business in their paper or on their website. This will allow your business free publicity instead of having to pay for advertising. They will also allow you to write your own press release, giving the public an overview of what your business can do for them. Contact your local newspaper and ask their representative about their free press release or go online at *www.bestwayclassifieds.com* or just Google free advertising online and you will be directed to sites. This will save you hundreds or thousands of dollars in advertising cost.

# SALES REPRESENTATIVE

(Contact Medical Supplier Customer Service)

When contacting each medical supply distributor's customer service department to setup your account, you will be asked where your business will be located. This is to put you in contact with the company's sales representative (Rep.) for your area. This is the person that you will be dealing with primarily for all your medical supply needs. This person will set your pricing for your equipment and supplies.

The sales rep. can also set special pricing on large quantity orders that you will get from your customers. This special pricing cannot be offered through customer service, so you will have to call your sales representative directly. This pricing will be significantly lower than the original pricing.

# WHAT CAN I SELL

The list of medical equipment and supplies is endless. As a new medical equipment and supply business owner, your goals are to provide your customers with the best products and services, and in a timely manner.

When entering into the business of selling medical equipment and supplies, and having very little to no knowledge of the business, I would recommend that you start out selling supplies that you are familiar with. Start out selling those supplies that are disposable (this will generate continuous orders on a month to month bases). Below is a list of equipment and supplies that are recurrent orders from month to month (or sooner). This list is a good start for those with no experience in the medical supply business.

| | |
|---|---|
| Gloves (Sterile, Non-Sterile) | Ace Bandage |
| Gowns (Patient, Isolation) | Biohazard Bags |
| Gauze | Trash Bags |
| Bandages | Mask |
| Sponges | Shoe Covers |
| Wipes | Crutches |
| Alcohol Prep Pads | Walkers |
| Under pads | Wheelchairs |
| Canes | Hand Sanitizer |

The list above is just a few of the everyday products that are being bought by these companies on a routine bases. You may see, or have even used these products yourself (common knowledge products). However, if you familiarize yourself with other medical products, your sells of the medical equipment and supplies will have no limits as to how far you can take your business

While conducting your business, you will occasionally be asked for products that you don't provide. Do not be so fast to say that you do not have it. Let your customer know that you will check to see if you can get it for them from the manufacturer. Then let your sales rep. know what's Product, and if they don't have it (do your best to find the product). Then notify your customer to let them know that you can or cannot get it for them (going the extra mile). This will go a long ways with your customers in building a good reputation and trust for your business.

Accommodating your customers' needs will take your business to a higher level, and your business name will be the first to come to mind when they need medical products.

# WHO DO I SELL TO AND WHAT DO I SAY?

## Who do I sell supplies to?

Below is just a short list of companies that buy medical supplies on a regular base.

Hospitals
Doctor's Office
Clinics
Nursing Homes
State Agencies (State Hospitals, Prisons, Health Departments, Mental Health Facilities, And State Procurement etc.) There is a pre registration that you will need to complete before qualifying to sell to state agencies. Contact your state small business office.
Schools, (Universities, private, public, etc)
Military
Home Health Agencies
Fire Department
Rescue squad
Federal Government: Must have your business registered on the Central Contracting Registration (CCR) prior to selling. Go online to: ccr.gov to register online
Group Homes
Assisted Living
Set up a Face book Business page (sell there)

**This is just a few of the many, many places that buy medical equipment and supplies.**

## What Do I Say?

When calling on these facilities, you want to ask for the person that's in charge or the one that handles the purchasing of their medical equipment and supplies. (It's usually an office manager or person who handles Procurement)

You would then introduce yourself, and ask if they would allow you the opportunity to come in and talk with the staff about your business and what you can offer to their company.

With State and Federal calling, you must first register your business as a vendor for that state. You would have to go to your state government website and register your business.

With the Federal Government you must go online @ ccr.gov and register your business. This has to be done in order to call on any federal agency to buy your products. (And they buy millions of dollars of product each year)

Be prepared when you go in to talk to these organizations. They are professionals and most have been in the business for years, and they know exactly what they want.

With the state and federal agencies, they are by law obligated to buy products and services from small businesses just like the one that you are starting. They are mandated to show that they have met their requirements each year that they have used a small business to provide a service or product to them.

# DROP SHIPPING

## (Contact Sales Representative)

When placing an order with some of the medical distributors you will be asked where they will be shipping your order.

Any order that you place and have shipped to an address (by the distributor) other than your place of business address is call drop shipping. For example, you get an order for 1000 boxes of gloves. You will then call your sales rep. or customer service to place your order. Customer service will confirm your order and ask you where we will be shipping. You will then give them your customer's address. At that point your order will be shipped directly from the distributor's warehouse to your customer. The order will never be in your possession, which eliminates you from stocking any supplies at your home.

Most of the distributors that provide this drop shipping service offer it free of charge. However, there are some that will charge you for providing this service, but only with a very small fee.

It will be your responsibility to confirm with your customer that their order is complete and to their satisfaction. Always try to the best of your ability to provide your customer with their product in a timely manner. If you say that the product will be there on Monday, try to have it to them prior to that day or on that day. It will also be your responsibility to make sure that your order is shipped from the distributor in a timely manner. Drop Shipping is great, but because you cannot inspect the product before it is shipped to your customers, it is necessary to stay on top of your distributors to be sure that your order is correct and shipped with no problems. (Call customer service or your sales rep. to confirm)

# MEDICAL SUPPLIER/DISTRIBUTOR COMPANIES

(Products Provided)

| Company | Products |
|---|---|
| Medline Industries | All |
| Drive Medical | Beds, Wheelchair, Crutches, Canes, etc. |
| Direct Supply | Beds, Wheelchair, Crutches, Canes, etc. |
| Gulf South Medical | All |
| Independence Medical | All |
| McKesson | All |
| Neil Medical | All |
| PSS (Physician Sales and Services) | All |
| Seca | Scales |
| Medplus Services | All |
| Moore Medical | All |
| Mercury Medical | All |
| Medegen | Bedside items (pitchers, basins, cups, etc.) |
| Invacare | Beds, Wheelchair, Walkers, Crutches, etc. |
| HD Medical Supply | Disposables |
| Market Lab | All |
| Healthcare Care Logistics | All |
| United Ad Labels | Medical Labels (Patient ID, Equip. etc.) |
| J. S. Spratley | Business Consultant Emergency Alert System |

# MEDICAL SUPPLIER/DISTRIBUTOR COMPANIES

### (Website)

| Company | Website |
| --- | --- |
| Medline Industries | www.medline.com |
| Drive Medical | www.drivemedicaldesign.com |
| Direct Supply | www.directsupply.net |
| Gulf South Medical | www.gsonline.com |
| Independence Medical | www.indemed.com |
| McKesson | www.mckesson.com |
| Neil Medical | www.neilmedical.com |
| PSS | www.mypss.com |
| Seca | www.seca-online.com |
| Medplus Services | www.medplusonline.com |
| Moore Medical | www.mooremedical.com |
| Mercury Medical | www.mercurymed.com |
| Medegen | www.medegen.com |
| Invacare | www.invacare.com |
| HD Medical Supply | www.hdmedicalsupply.com |
| Market Lab | www.marketlabinc.com |
| Healthcare Care Logistics | www.healthcarelogistics.com |
| United Ad Labels | www.unitedadlabel.com |
| J. S. Spratley | 770-557-8631 |

# MEDICAL SUPPLIER/DISTRIBUTOR COMPANIES

### (Phone List)

| Company | Phone Number |
| --- | --- |
| Medline Industries | 800-633-5463 |
| Drive Medical | 877-224-0946 + 1 |
| Direct Supply | 800-634-7328 |
| Gulf South Medical | 800-347-2456 |
| Independence Medical | 800-860-8027 |
| McKesson | 888-822-8111 |
| Neil Medical | 800-735-9111 |
| PSS (Physician Sales and Services) | 904-332-3000 |
| Seca | 800-542-7322 |
| Medplus Services | 877-436-5378 |
| Moore Medical | 800-234-1464 |
| Mercury Medical | 800-237-6418 |
| Medegen | 800-233-1987 |
| Invacare | 800-333-6900 |
| HD Medical Supply | 404-919-6338 |
| Market Lab | 800-237-3604 |
| Health Care Logistics | 800-848-1633 |
| United Add Labels | 800-992-575 |
| J. S. Spratley | 770-557-8631 |

# HELPFUL SITES

The list below gives you websites that can be used to enhance and grow your business.

**Websites:** *www.wix.com*
*www.yola.com*
*www.webstarts.com*
*www.jimdo.com*
*www.tiptopwebsite.com*

**Advertising:** Local news paper (press release)
Face-book Advertising (*www.facebook.com/ads*)
Amazon Advertising (*www.amazonservices.com/productads*)

**Phones:** (*www.phonebooth.com/free-business-voip*)
(*www.evoice.com*)
(*www.googlevoice.com*)

**Business Cards:** Google "Free Business Cards" (Allows you to do it Yourself)

These sites listed are just a few among the numerous sites listed online. If you Google these sites, you can find many more, For example; Google "free websites" or "free Advertising" or "free phone numbers" all of which will give you options to choose from.

# CALCULATION OF YOUR START-UP COST;

| Description | Cost |
|---|---|
| Zoning | 00.00 |
| Register Business Name | 10.00 |
| Business License | 00.00 |
| Tax ID/EIN | 00.00 |
| Business Bank Account | 100.00 |
| Business Insurance | 00.00 |
| Fax | 00.00 |
| Business Cards | 00.00 |
| Credit Card processing | 00.00 |
| Recordkeeping Journal | 5.00 |
| Press Release | 00.00 |
| Board of Pharmacy License | 175.00 (may vary) |

**When you add these numbers the total of your start-up is less than $300.00, for a business that could earn you millions!**

# DID YOU REMEMBER

(Start-up Checklist)

____ Zoning Requirements

____ Register Business Name

____ Business License

____ Tax Identification/Employer Identification Number (EIN)

____ Business Bank Account

____ Tax (Register State and Local)

____ Other License (Your State Board of Pharmacy)

____ Business Insurance

**The list above is what you will need to do to be legally ready to do business.**

**The list below is what needs to be done, but can wait.**

____ Business Tools (Computer, Phone, Fax, Website)

____ Business Material (Business Cards/Fliers)

____ Payment (Merchant Service, Pay Pal, Credit Card. Check)

____ Recordkeeping/Bookkeeping (QuickBooks or Journal)

____ Medical Supplier Companies (Customer Service)

____ Privacy Act (HIPAA.Gov)

____ Press Release

# MEDICAL GLOVE MARKET RESEARCH

### Global Disposable Medical Gloves Market to Reach $3.4 Billion by 2015, According to a New Report by Global Industry Analysts, Inc.

GIA announces the release of a comprehensive global report on the Disposable Medical Gloves markets. The global market for Disposable Medical Gloves is projected to reach US$3.4 billion by the year 2015. Factors contributing to the rise in consumption levels include healthcare reforms in several countries, and rising emphasis on health, occupational safety and hygiene among end-users in medical, dental and service industries.

Though the healthcare industry felt the lingering effects of adverse economic conditions in recent times largely due to rising capital costs and unfavorable reimbursement scenario, the disposable medical gloves market however survived the crisis primarily attributed to the indispensable use of gloves in the healthcare industry. The year 2009, witnessed a significant increase in disposable gloves sales on account of the H1N1 pandemic. Further, rise in personal and occupational hygiene standards amid outbreak of various infections such as avian flu, SARS and HIV continued to sustain market growth in recent years. There exists immense opportunities for growth in the global medical gloves market given the fact that dozens of pairs of medical gloves are utilized in a single day in hospitals and laboratorial settings around the world. The US and Europe dominate the global Disposable Medical Gloves market, as stated by the new market research report on Disposable Medical Gloves market. Driven by improvements in healthcare sector and the Rising standard of living together with the increasing importance of controlling cross contamination and infections in hospitals and clinics have led to increased demand for latex surgical gloves in markets such as China and India.

Examination gloves that primarily aid in the prevention of microbial contamination of hands of the health care workers during various routine hospital procedures, represents the largest product segment. Currently, the growing awareness of latex induced side effects in surgical patients, and allergy in regular users have led to a major market shift from powdered latex to powder free latex, and synthetic medical gloves. Surgical gloves form the fastest growing product category.

13th of January 2011 @ 09:00 | Source: PR Web

Home » Kalorama Is A Leading Global Publisher Of Market Studies On Heal . . . Channel » Press Release » Global Disposable Medical Gloves Market to Reach US$3.4 Billion . . .

{PR Web via Bio Portfolio}

26888864R00029

Made in the USA
Lexington, KY
28 October 2013